The Hormone Reset Diet for Women:

Lose Weight Quickly and Safely for Life with the Hormone Reset Diet Plan

KARA AIMER

CONTENTS

INTRODUCTION

Most women experience unusual changes in their bodies and accept such as something that "naturally happens." However, some women choose to fight and get back what time has taken from them. These are the women who were tired of getting constant mood swings, feeling tired all the time, not being able to get a good night's rest, not being able to enjoy sex, gaining unwelcome pounds, and feeling old.

There's so much power contained in the body of a woman – the power of multitasking, the power of visual acuity, the power of intuition, and so much more. What comes with that power, however, can ironically leave a woman feeling powerless.

Through time, scientists noticed a lot of overlap between the symptoms of aging and the symptoms of hormonal imbalance. Some of the problems women with hormonal imbalance often experience include the inability to lose weight, fatigue, low quality sleep, mood swings, anxiety, depression, brain fog, and random rush of warmth to certain parts of your body.

Notice how these symptoms of hormonal imbalance are rather similar to the things aging women often experience. A side-by-side comparison easily shows you that one could have caused the other, or both are really the same thing. If you've been experiencing even just one of these symptoms, you may need to take steps to help your hormone levels go back to normal.

Fortunately, there are simple ways to restore your body's optimal hormone levels and one of them is by hacking it using hormone reset techniques. This isn't just for women beyond the age of 40. Studies show that because of the prolonged stress induced by a hectic lifestyle, women even at the age of 18 may already experience hormonal imbalance. There's always a need to manage hormone level whether one is in her teens or in her eighties.

What a lot of people don't realize is that hormones control a great deal of what's happening inside a woman's body. Basically, hormones dictate how fast you can lose weight, how happy you can be, how much stress you can handle, and so much more. Hormone reset is basically the holy grail of anti-aging that isn't so well explored compared to cosmetics.

Hormones are the key to keeping one's body balanced, but since women have much more complicated hormones than men, there is a need for a good battle plan.

By getting this book, you're already on your first step to getting your life back. This book will help you feel good and look good using the latest hormonal balance techniques

HORMONES: AN INTRODUCTION

Everyone experienced stumbling down at some point. However, there is one common denominator in all these experiences: one assesses what made her fall, learns from her experiences, gets up and remembers to avoid whatever has made her stumble. In this chapter, you'll have an overview about hormones, with estrogen as the focal point since it is one of the most important hormones you'll have to keep in check.

What are hormones?

The human body is like a company, with different departments handling specific tasks, all vital for the company to thrive. Hormones act as messengers, telling departments to speed up, slow down, or stop whatever they're doing, in order to keep them in sync with each other.

What is estrogen?

Estrogen is a hormone that primarily regulates a woman's reproductive development including menstruation. It also regulates other parts of the body, including the brain, heart, breast, skin, hair, etc. Estrogen helps keep your body temperature stable, which is good for your brain because this also allows you to think properly.

It also regulates the amount of cholesterol produced by the liver, which is beneficial for your heart. A healthy level of estrogen is also good for your ovaries because it helps them develop. When it is ready, the hormone helps indicate the start of the menstrual cycle. Should you choose to conceive, estrogen also helps the uterus give the developing fetus the nourishment it needs. It also aids in keeping your bones dense and strong.

What happens when your hormone levels plummet?

Stable hormone levels keep you happy and healthy because all of your organs know what they are supposed to do and can, therefore, function efficiently. Your ovaries are the largest producers of estrogen and progesterone, both of which are important hormones that control the reproductive system. However, in order to regulate the amount of estrogen, progesterone, and testosterone in your body, the pituitary gland produces luteinizing and follicle-stimulating hormones.

Once you reach the menopausal stage, some parts of your body, specifically the ovaries, become less responsive to the luteinizing and follicle-stimulating hormones. This can cause your estrogen levels to fall as well. The problem is that hormones are interconnected; a huge decline in estrogen levels can easily affect other hormones working to keep your body stable. Here is how plummeting hormone levels affect your body:

No monthly periods - Probably, the most obvious change during menopause is the absence of a monthly period, so a woman will no longer being able to conceive.

Hot flashes - Since estrogen helps keep your body temperature stable, if not enough is produced, you will most likely experience a strange rush of warmth in different parts of your body. A lot of women report feeling hot flashes on their face, neck, chest, or back that last from seconds to perhaps an hour.

Vaginal dryness and thinning - Since estrogen helps keep your vagina well lubricated and protected, lack of it will cause dryness and even painful intercourse.

Mood swings - Moodiness is a well-known side effect of menopause because of the sharp decrease in estrogen production. Basically, the brain conks out because it does not get the same amount of estrogen that it was used to getting. This causes you to feel happy one second and then angry after just a few seconds.

Fatigue - Fluctuating hormone levels force your body to spend energy trying to keep things stable. Eventually, this causes you to feel drained, angry and grumpy.

Memory loss. Estrogen helps your brain think straight and even multitask. A decline in estrogen levels also means a decline in focus. When you can't focus, you are bound to forget things easily, especially when you try to multitask.

Summary

You have already been given a quick overview of hormones, specifically estrogen, and how these can make or break your day depending on how much your body produces them. In the next chapter, you will learn more about different hormones and how they affect your mood, energy, sex life, and other aspects of your everyday life. You'll be taught how to rebalance your hormones using simple yet effective hormone reset techniques.

HORMONE REBALANCING ACT

Before getting back up, you have to know what caused your fall. This chapter will tell you more about the important hormones you need to keep in check, what happens when they are out of balance and are unstable, and how you can rebalance them with simple lifestyle hacks. Let us go through each important hormone in detail:

Hormones for Energy and Weight Control

Cortisol - In the time of dinosaurs and unfurnished caves, there were plenty of dangerous predators that roamed free. A person you've met a while ago could have been turned to dinosaur food a few seconds after. The human body has adapted to the dangers of the prehistoric times by releasing a stress hormone known as cortisol when confronted by a life-or-death situation.

In doing so, your heart beats faster, you think much more clearly, and basically you become wonder woman for a few seconds. However, after this brief moment of super strength, the body feels exhausted and will need to replenish the rapidly depleted energy.

This system of energy expenditure worked quite well in the past, as it helped the human race survive, but right now, the body releases cortisol even for non-life-threatening situations, like working for a terrible boss, spending hours in traffic, etc. What happens when what was initially meant to be short bursts of energy expenditure are turned into long triathlons of energy expenditure? The body will start to fail in performing its functions and you'll pretty soon feel tired and spent all the time.

Protocol. A lot of women put off cardio exercise because they feel too tired. Studies show, however, that doing cardio and weight training at least three times a week will reduce the amount of cortisol released by the body and will, therefore, help your energy levels remain stable throughout the day. Get a gym membership if you can, since gym trainers can give you more specialized exercises that fit your body type. By exercising three times a week, you get your energy back while getting a lot closer to wearing those skinny jeans.

Melatonin – The hormone that is known to help regulate the reproductive cycle and give you that quality, restorative sleep is released at night when it is completely dark. Your body produces a lot of melatonin usually in the wee hours of the morning. However, when something prevents your body from fully falling asleep, like bluish light sources or caffeine, your pineal gland may not produce enough melatonin. This will cause you to wake up feeling groggy, grumpy, and grouchy.

Also, when your body does not get enough melatonin for long periods of time, you get a higher risk of getting cancer and diabetes. Lastly, low melatonin levels can cause obesity.

Protocol. Make sure that your bedroom is pitch-black when you go to sleep. If you can't completely prevent sources of light from entering your room, invest in an eye mask instead. Around three hours before going to sleep, do not watch television or avoid doing anything on the computer or on your smartphone. These items emit blue light, which is known to affect melatonin release even after a few hours of getting exposed to them.

If you really need to use the computer before going to bed, you may want to try f.lux, a free program that adjusts the color of your monitor so that at night, the screen becomes less bluish and more yellowish. Lastly, avoid sleeping with your bra and other restrictive clothing on. When your body is in an uncomfortable state, it reduces its melatonin production by almost half.

Thyroid - Do you have friends who do not seem to gain weight no matter how much they eat? They have their thyroid glands to thank for that. The thyroid hormones control how fast your metabolism is and how much energy you can spend. With long-term stress, bad diets, and thyroid diseases, however, the thyroid gland may malfunction and cause you to gain or lose too much weight, have too much or too little energy, etc.

Protocol. Lab tests are the best way to find out if you have a thyroid problem or not. However, if the problem isn't too serious, you can simply take high quality bioavailable multivitamins (a shortcut to knowing if a multivitamin is bioavailable or not is by making sure that vitamin B12 is labeled as methyl-cobalamin and not cyanocobalamin). In most cases, however, it is best to consult a medical doctor if you think that you have a thyroid problem.

Hormones for Appetite Control

Leptin - Do you tend to get 2nd, 3rd, or even 4th servings because you don't get full easily? Blame leptin; it is the hormone that suppresses your appetite and gives you that satisfied feeling when you are full. If your leptin levels are out of control then you are bound to overeat.

Protocol. A lot of times, sugar has been the culprit for low leptin levels, which is why a lot of people who tend to overeat are actually sweet tooth's. In the next chapter, we're going to talk about meals that will satisfy your cravings for sweets while helping your body regulate leptin production.

Ghrelin - Being the partner-in-crime of leptin, ghrelin is the hormone responsible for telling you to raid the fridge for something to eat when you're hungry. The key phrase here is "when you are hungry", and not "when you are bored". Unfortunately, if your leptin levels are out of control, ghrelin ends up mixing up these two phrases; therefore, causing you to eat out of boredom.

Protocol. Your ghrelin levels should go back to normal as soon as your leptin levels are stable. This basically means cutting down on foods filled with refined sugar. Don't fret, though; the recipes in the next chapter will show you just how tasty and easy-to-prepare healthy foods are.

Hormones for Love, Sex and Happiness

Serotonin - Known as the happiness hormone, serotonin is created by your intestines coming from the carbohydrates you take in. In the morning, melatonin levels drop to make way for serotonin. This means that when sunlight touches your face, melatonin production is dramatically reduced to make you feel less sleepy, and serotonin production is dramatically increased to make you more alert.

Also, it has been noted that serotonin is one of the major factors that allow a woman to multitask. Low levels of serotonin often mean less energy, crappy mood swings, and the loss of the ability to multitask.

Protocol. A lot of women with low levels of serotonin turn out to be participating in some kind of low-carb diet, like the Atkins diet. Remember that your body needs an adequate amount of carbohydrates and tryptophan in order to create serotonin, and a lot of low-carb foods don't have these vital ingredients. The next chapter will discuss foods that will help your body create the serotonin it needs while helping you stay lean.

Oxytocin - Known as the love hormone, oxytocin is released whenever you touch someone you love, whether that someone is a friend or a lover. This hormone is responsible for that powerful rush of euphoria you get towards people you love. Do you remember the last time you had a crush on someone, and it ended up being your main thought of the day/week/month? Oxytocin becomes rather invasive at times; it is capable of making your brain forget other things when you are in love and is, therefore, dangerous if not regulated.

However, the problem usually is not the excess of oxytocin, but the lack of it. With too little oxytocin, more fights are bound to happen, along with more feelings of loneliness and isolation even within a relationship.

Protocol. Since oxytocin is released when you touch someone you love, the best way to boost oxytocin release is by snuggling with your special somebody, whether it's a person or a pet. If you're living alone, studies show that daydreaming about someone you love can also help boost oxytocin production. However, the best way to boost oxytocin turned out to be sex, as oxytocin production was overdriven before and after an orgasm.

Testosterone - While normally considered a guy's sex hormone, testosterone plays an important role in a woman's body as well. It helps you burn fat and build muscle. It revs up your metabolism and boosts your sex drive. The amount of testosterone produced in a woman's body is miniscule in comparison to the amount of testosterone produced in a man's body, which means that a slight reduction in testosterone level for a woman means a sudden drop of energy, mood, and sex drive. Slight excess, on the other hand, means the appearance of unsightly facial hair and other stuff you don't want.

Protocol. Just like cortisol, you need a good exercise routine to keep your testosterone levels in check, along with the right diet, which we'll get into later. However, some women get irregular testosterone spikes that a simple lifestyle change cannot fix. In this case, it is best to find a good gynecologist to help you sort things out with testosterone.

Estrogen - We've talked about this in great detail back in Chapter 1. Without a healthy amount of estrogen in your system, a lot of things can easily take place - from irritability to anxiety, to depression.

Protocol. Being one of the most important hormones to keep in check, it makes sense that your best form of defense is to eat the right types of food. In the next chapter, we're going to talk about meals that can help your body control its estrogen levels and other hormone levels as well.

EATING YOUR WAY BACK TO PERFECT HEALTH

What you eat greatly affects how certain hormones are produced and absorbed in your body. In the previous chapter, you may have noticed that apart from lack of exercise and thyroid and ovular diseases, a lot of hormonal imbalances are caused by an imbalanced nutrient intake coming from a bad diet. A lot of women starve themselves on low-carb, low-everything diets that actually end up messing their metabolism and causing all kinds of wreckage on their hormones.

Fortunately, eating your way back to perfect health does not have to be painfully tasteless and dull. Here are some of the best recipes you can try for the perfect balance of taste and good health:

Breakfast

Are you in a hurry to start your day? Ditch the high-sugar cereal and opt for a more delicious, filling, and healthier meal instead using these recipes:

Chocolate Almond Smoothie

Ingredients:
¼ cup of instant oatmeal
2 tablespoons of almond butter
1 tablespoon of cacao nibs
1 cup unsweetened coconut juice
2 servings of whey protein powder
Stevia (depends on how sweet you want your shake to be)

Instructions:

1.   Put them all in a blender and blend for about a minute or two. Save half for your next breakfast or share it with another person.

Nutty Peach and Blueberry Smoothie

Ingredients:
½ cup of peach
½ cup of blueberries
3 Brazil nuts
1 teaspoon vanilla extract
½ cup butter lettuce
1 teaspoon maca
½ cup of Almond milk

Instructions:

1.   Put all the ingredients into the blender and add water as needed.

2.   Blend for about a minute or two. This recipe can serve two people.

Avocado Smoothie

Ingredients:
1 peeled avocado without the seed
2 servings of whey protein powder
1 banana
2 plum tomatoes
1 cup of spinach

Instructions:

1.   Put all the ingredients into the blender and add water as needed.

2.   Blend for about two minutes to three minutes. This recipe can serve two people.

Blueberry Yogurt Smoothie

Ingredients:
1 cup blueberries
1 cup yogurt

1 banana
2 cups of whey protein powder
1 tablespoon chia seeds

Instructions:
1.   Put all ingredients into the blender and blend for about a minute or two. This can serve two people.

Creamy Cherry Smoothie

Ingredients:
½ cup of cherries
1 teaspoon vanilla extract
¼ cup of instant oatmeal
2 cups of whey protein powder
1 cup natural unsweetened coconut juice
2 tablespoons of olive oil or flaxseed oil

Instructions:
1.   Put all ingredients into the blender and blend for about a minute or two. This can serve two people.
2.   Add stevia as desired.

Lunch

A healthy breakfast perks you up for the morning. A healthy lunch perks you up for the afternoon. Here are some yummy and healthy options to avoid that afternoon crash:

Chicken Lettuce Wraps

Ingredients:
1 boneless and skinless chicken breast (cooked and diced)
¼ cup Greek yogurt
6 romaine lettuce leaves (large)
2 teaspoons of extra virgin olive oil
1 tablespoon of grinded red onion
1 diced green apple
¼ cup diced cucumber
¼ cup diced red bell pepper

Salt and pepper as desired

Instructions:
1.   Put everything except for the lettuce in a large bowl and mix well.
2.   Let it chill for at least an hour (preferably overnight to help flavors combine).
3.   Place mixture into the lettuce leaves and wrap 'em up. Enjoy!

Salmon Teriyaki

Ingredients:
1½ lb. salmon filet (about 6 pieces)
1 teaspoon of toasted sesame oil
2 tablespoons of Japanese rice wine (mirin)
¼ cup soy sauce
1 lb. asparagus sliced to chunks with ends removed

Instructions:
1.   Place salmon in a large bowl.
2.   Mix the Japanese rice wine with the soy sauce and sesame oil in order to create a marinade.
3.   Mix the salmon and asparagus with the marinade and refrigerate for at least half an hour (preferably overnight).
4.   Preheat oven to broil.
5.   Remove the salmon and asparagus from the bowl and place them on a cooking sheet.
6.   Broil until salmon starts to flake and the asparagus softens (usually about 3-5 minutes)
7.   Serve with organic brown rice. Enjoy!

Spicy Chicken

Ingredients:
2 cubed boneless and skinless chicken breasts
1 can of white beans
4 cups of chicken broth
½ teaspoon of ground cumin
1 teaspoon of dried oregano
4 oz. of diced mushrooms
½ diced green pepper
½ diced orange pepper

¼ teaspoon black pepper
¼ teaspoon garlic salt
1 chopped onion
1 tablespoon extra virgin olive oil
2 minced garlic cloves
1 chopped and seeded jalapeño pepper
¾ cup of diced celery
2 cups of diced carrots
1 sliced avocado
1 cup of chopped kale

Instructions:
1.   Add salt and pepper to the chicken.
2.   Fry the chicken until it turns golden brown. Use medium heat.
3.   Add in the garlic, jalapeño, mushrooms, onions, peppers and stir for about a minute or two.
4.   Add the ground cumin and dried oregano and cook until the chicken turns golden brown and the vegetables soften.
5.   Transfer everything to a slow cooker.
6.   Mix ½ cup of chicken broth with a cup of mashed white beans.
7.   Add the mashed beans and chicken broth to the slow cooker.
8.   Mix in the rest of the chicken broth, white beans, diced carrots, diced celery, and kale to the slow cooker.
9.   Cover and cook under low heat until the chicken is soft enough.
10.   Stir and add sliced avocado.
11.   Serve with Brown Rice.
12.   Share with three other people or store the rest for other days. Enjoy!

Dinner

After a tiring day at work, it is nice to come home to a delicious and healthy meal. However, it is best to consume foods that the body can easily digest since the last thing you want is an overworking digestive system while you sleep.

These two recipes do not contain beef, pork, or any other ingredients that take a long time for the body to digest so that your hunger is satisfied without making you feel sluggish in the morning.

Scrumptious Chicken Salad

Ingredients:
3 poached and shredded chicken breasts
½ sliced head of green cabbage
1 cup of chopped cilantro leaves
1 shallot
2 shredded carrots
2 sliced stalks of celery
2 sliced red bell peppers
3 sliced green onions
1/3 cup of sliced, toasted almonds
3 tablespoons soy sauce
¼ cup avocado oil
¼ cup sesame oil
3 tablespoons of white vinegar
Peeled and sliced small piece of ginger

Instructions:
1.   Mix the chicken and vegetables together
2.   Blend the oil, vinegar, sauce, and other ingredients for the dressing.
3.   Share with three other people or store for another day. Enjoy!

Savory Rice with Vegetables

Ingredients:
1 cup of brown rice
2 cups of vegetable broth
1 cup of quartered button mushrooms
½ cup of sliced red pepper
2 teaspoons of sesame oil
½ cup of diced white onion
1 teaspoon of grated ginger
1 tablespoon of miso paste
½ cup of sliced zucchini
1/3 cup of pine nuts

Instructions:
1.   Rinse the cup of brown rice only once then soak for 30 minutes in a 2-quart saucepan.
2.   Add in the broth and let it simmer for about half an hour. Make sure the saucepan is covered.

3.   Add the sesame oil to a non-stick heavy-bottomed saucepan.

4.   Sauté the diced white onion, sliced zucchini, sliced red pepper, grated ginger, and quartered button mushrooms until the vegetables are tender.

5.   Add in the miso paste and pine nuts and continue cooking for about another minute.

6.   Mix the rice and vegies.

7.   Share with three other people or store for another day. Enjoy!

SUPPLEMENTS

In the past, our ancestors got all the nutrients they needed from the sun, the sea, and all the natural sources of food that surround them. Long-term stress was basically non-existent as they live in a world with no bosses, taxes, bills, and other complicated forms of stressful activities we have come to terms with.

Since our living conditions have now completely changed, it is likely that we no longer meet our nutritional needs from the foods we eat and the environment we live in. Here are some of the best supplements known to help your body maintain stable hormone levels:

Maca – You have seen this ingredient in some of the recipes we have talked about. If you are not adding this to your diet, you'll definitely want this in your medicine cabinet, as it is known to prevent PMS while giving your skin a healthy glow and keeping your hormones in check.

Magnesium - If you have been experiencing low-quality sleep, you may be low in magnesium. Adequate amounts of magnesium will help your body release the right kinds of hormones when you sleep (melatonin) and when you wake up (serotonin).

Vitamin D - Vitamin D helps your hormones behave. The best form of Vitamin D is from the sun, but if you live in an area where the sun only comes out a few times a year, opt for a high-quality multivitamin instead.

Coconut oil. Did you know that you could use coconut oil for coffee or tea? By doing so, you help your body produce the necessary hormones while reducing inflammation and keeping itself free from bacteria and microbes. Simply blend a tablespoon of coconut oil with ¼ teaspoon of vanilla, 1 teaspoon unsalted butter, and stevia as desired, together with your favorite coffee or tea and you will have an amazing energy-boosting hormone-balancing drink to help you conquer the day.

GENERAL GUIDELINES IN CHOOSING WHAT TO EAT

Sometimes, it is just impossible to go with a completely healthy home cooked meal. The grocery store also offers a variety of junk foods, some of them pretending to be healthy. Here are some guidelines to help you stay healthy even with a plethora of junk foods surrounding you:

Avoid foods with ingredients you can't pronounce. This advice has been passed down through generations of organic-lovers. In most cases, hard to pronounce ingredients are chemically synthesized and may cause unwelcome side effects to the body. For example, aspartame, a common sugar substitute, is considered an excitotoxin, which basically means that it wreaks havoc to your brain.

Another well-known excitotoxin is MSG, which stands for monosodium glutamate. MSG is widely used because of its ability to make even the blandest foods tasty and delicious. However, a lot of people have experienced headaches, brain fog, and other cognitive problems after being exposed to foods high in MSG.

MSG can also be disguised as hydrolyzed vegetable protein, natural flavors, or even just spices. These ingredients contain up to 40% MSG.

It always helps to be on guard when selecting organic and natural foods. Choose ones that have the most pronounceable ingredients and you are more likely to be purchasing the right kind of food.

Cut down on caffeinated beverages. Caffeinated beverages may be able to give you that quick boost of energy, but in a few hours, that feeling will quickly fade. Because your body eventually becomes tolerant to caffeine, you start to need more than a cup of coffee to stay awake.

Soon enough, you start drinking more than three cups of coffee a day, and this wreaks havoc on your endocrine system and causes the dreaded "adrenal fatigue." When this happens, no amount of coffee can save your sudden energy crash and you will end up feeling horrible the next few days.

It is not advisable to go cold turkey especially if you are working a 9-5 job, so the key is to slowly reduce the amount of caffeine you are consuming until you eventually reach just one cup of coffee a day. If you are craving for a hot beverage, here are some herbal teas that can help boost your energy levels naturally:

Rooibos tea - Generally known as a good coffee replacement, rooibos can offer a clean energy boost with only positive side effects, like boosting your immune system, getting rid of those nasty stomach cramps and headaches, and helping you get some shut eye.

Ginseng tea - Ginseng is one of the most well-known herbs that can help you fight off stress and fatigue that comes from the most common stress triggers.

Gingko Biloba tea - Commonly known as the 'smart herb', gingko biloba can help improve and regulate blood flow to the brain, which can give you razor-sharp focus and an amazing memory. It can perform especially well when combined with ginseng.

Licorice tea - Licorice is one of the few herbs that can fix a wide range of problems - from fatigue to depression, to unstable blood sugar levels. This is a great tea to have in your desk especially if you just had a meal packed with sugar.

Green Tea - Green tea contains a small amount of caffeine, so you can even use this to replace your morning cup of coffee. What makes this a better alternative for coffee is the fact that it contains much less caffeine. It also has an ingredient called L-theanine, which counteracts the jitters and jumpiness caffeine is known for.

Avoid oil with manmade fats. Vegetable oil, canola oil, soybean oil, and peanut oil contain high levels of polyunsaturated fats, which are highly unstable and easily cause problems when your body uses them to create and repair cells.

Make sure that you opt for healthier oils instead, like olive oil (that you should never ever heat) and coconut oil.

Read the labels word for word. A lot of food companies try to trick customers into thinking that what they are selling are all-natural by inserting some weasel words into their products. Here are some of the misleading labels you should be aware of:

All natural - Just because something says "all natural" in the label does not mean it follows the generally accepted meaning of 'natural'. Since the Food and Drug Administration does not have a strict ruling on what types of food could have an "all-natural" label, any types of food that do not have artificial flavors, colors, or synthetic substances can be considered "all natural."

Some companies even argue that products with high fructose corn syrup (a substance you really want to cut out of your diet) come from corn, which means that they are healthy (which is really not the case).

Multigrain or Made with Whole Grain - Healthy types of bread, pancakes, etc. are made from whole grain, not with whole grain. Multigrain and other products "made from whole grain" are often stripped of fiber and other important nutrients that whole grain products offer. Opt for products only with the labels, 100% whole grain or whole grain.

No sugar added - This is another tactic food companies use to trick dieting people to consume their sugar-loaded treats without feeling guilty. Note that no sugar added simply means that they haven't added extra sugar to their products. Fruits and other products naturally contain sugar and, therefore, do not disqualify products from having that extremely misleading label.

Sugar-free - Be extremely cautious when buying foods, especially sweets, claiming not to have sugar. Sugar replacements tend to cause more sugar cravings and cognitive decline in the long run, so keep in mind that oftentimes, it is better to get the regular version of a sugary product and shed the excess sugar with exercise.

Gluten-free - Gluten-free products are quickly becoming a trend, but unless you have the rare celiac disease or are intolerant of gluten, you won't really benefit from these kinds of products. Gluten-free is really more of a buzz word that tends to trick a lot of people into paying more for something they do not even need, so don't buy a product just because you see a "Gluten-free" label.

Made with Real Fruit - Just like the "made with whole grain" facade, products that claim to be made with real fruit often contains insignificant amounts of fruit and loads of artificial flavoring and sugar. Since companies do not have to disclose the percentage of their ingredients, there is no way to tell how much real fruit is in a certain package.

Check the order of the ingredients. A nifty trick to check the most abundant ingredient in a product is to see how the ingredients are listed. The most abundant ingredient in a product is usually listed first and the least abundant ingredient is usually listed last. Beware when you see sugar as the first ingredient; it usually means you're looking at junk food.

Avoid eating pork and beef for dinner. It is always advisable to stick to fish, veggies and lean chicken meat, but if you really need to satisfy your cravings for pork and beef, opt to eat them only during breakfast or lunch; pork and beef tire out your digestive system and will cause you to need more hours of sleep to feel refreshed in the morning.

SUMMARY

The tips, techniques and recipes mentioned in this chapter serve to debunk the myth that healthy foods taste rather dull while filling in nutritional gaps you may have. In the first few days, your taste buds are going to adapt to the different flavors you are experiencing, but don't fret; in a few weeks, you will have "educated" taste buds that will no longer crave for junk food and other hormone-production-disrupting foods.

Feel free to add, replace or remove ingredients as necessary. Everyone has different tastes, so keep playing with the proportions of the ingredients until you find the perfect recipe that works for you. There are plenty of healthy and delicious recipes online for you to try, and with this chapter as your starting point, you can now eat your way back to perfect health.

CONCLUSION

There are lots of expensive hormone therapies available, but a lot of times, the answer is not found in cold hospital rooms but in the things you do and the foods you eat. Every woman's body has different reactions to the tips and techniques mentioned in this book, so feel free to make the necessary adjustments to make this book work for you.

Remember to take things slow. Your body may experience a shock if you apply all of the hormone-reset techniques at once. You can start replacing your meals by using the new recipes two to three times a week then adding a few days as you get used to healthier foods. As for exercising, if you have never gone to a gym in your life, you may need a longer recovery time after your first few gym visits. If your body is still sore after a whole day of rest, add another day or two until the soreness disappears.

While some women are able to abandon their bad habits within a week, it typically takes about 21 days to make a new habit stick. You may not get some habits to stick on the first try, but keep going. The results are worth it. 21 days of pain is a small price to pay for staying young, healthy, happy, and beautiful for the years to come.

I hope this book has been an eye-opener for you and was able to help you get your life back on track. These tips and techniques are only the tips of the iceberg; this book simply serves to show you how amazingly complex a woman's body is and how you can hack yours to get more energy, think clearly, focus better, and much more!

Remember that the discovery of your own body should not end with this book. Stay hungry for knowledge and keep finding new ways to thrive in your hectic lifestyle, and your body will reward you by giving you a radiant glow, a reduction in wrinkles, a flat stomach, consistent energy, and a boosted mood to start and end the day.

Finally, if you enjoyed this book, please click below to share your thoughts and post a positive review on Amazon. I would greatly appreciate your support!

Thank you and good luck!

Kara Aimer

ADDITIONAL RESOURCES

Please point your web browser to **www.plaid-enterprises.com** for more related resources, my full bibliography and to grab your FREE book!